Natural Treatments for
DEPRESSION

USING ST. JOHN'S WORT, 5-HTP, VALERIAN AND OTHER THERAPIES TO NATURALLY OVERCOME DEPRESSION

C.M. Hawken

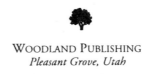

WOODLAND PUBLISHING
Pleasant Grove, Utah

CONTENTS

NATURAL TREATMENTS FOR DEPRESSION

DEPRESSION—AN OVERVIEW

Depression is a disorder that affects millions of people, both in the United States and worldwide. It is probably the most common psychiatric complaint given to doctors, and has been described by physicians as far back as the time of Hippocrates, who called it "melancholia." According to one recently published report, depression affects nearly 17 percent of all Americans for the length of their lives (Linde, et al. 253). It takes many forms, but is usually marked by sadness, inactivity and heightened self-depreciation. Hopelessness and pessimism are often common symptoms, as are lowered self-esteem, reduced energy and vitality, and loss of the overall capability to enjoy one's existence.

How depression affects people varies widely from person to person. Depression may be short-term, or may occur repeatedly at short intervals. It may be somewhat permanent, mild or severe, acute or chronic. And who does depression most affect? Rates of incidence are higher among women than men (for varying reasons, some not totally understood). Men are more at risk of suffering from depression as they age, while a woman's peak age for experiencing depression is usually between the ages of 35-45.

Depression is caused by many things—it could come about because of childhood traumas, other physical disorders or because of stressful life events—but more and more, doctors and scientists are pointing to a variety of factors, not one sole cause, as usually being the culprit. These can include overly stressful situations at work or home, biochemical processes, diet, other illness(es), drug use, and others. For instance, it is known that defective regulation of the release of one or more naturally occurring amines in the brain—particularly norepinephrine, serotonin and dopamine—leads to reduced quantities or reduced activity of these chemicals in the brain, bringing on the depressed mood for most sufferers. Other health experts are pointing to underlying, yet known, health conditions like diabetes or cancer as bringing on depression. And yet other experts point to a simple cause—lack of exercise—that can easily relieve, if not completely eradicate, depression symptoms.

TYPES OF DEPRESSION

When talking of depression, it may be sometimes difficult to understand what exactly constitutes depression. Certainly life presents us with situations, events and time periods that can make us feel "down" and perhaps even desperate and hopeless. But these feelings are normal in certain circumstances. It is only when these episodes become extreme, last for long periods, or overcome a person's life do we typically make the diagnosis of depression.

There are several different classes of depression, but for our purposes here, when we refer to "depression," we are talking about mild to moderate levels of depression, a condition often referred to as dysthemia, which is the most common type of depression. The other major forms of depression have their own labels: major depression (bi-polar disorders, manic depression), post-stroke depression, seasonal affective disorder (SAD), and post-partum depression.

Clinical Depression (Dysthemia)

According to the American Psychiatric Association, the symptoms of clinical depression, or dysthemia, include the following:

• Poor appetite with weight loss, or increased appetite with weight gain
• Physical hyperactivity or inactivity
• Loss of interest or pleasure in usual activities, or decrease in sexual drive
• Insomnia or hypersomnia (excessive sleeping)
• Feelings of worthlessness, self-reproach or inappropriate guilt

- Diminished ability to think or concentrate
- Recurrent thoughts of death or suicide

According to the APA's manual, *Diagnostic and Statistical Manual of Mental Disorders* (DSM-III), one must experience five of these eight symptoms to definitely qualify as being depressed. Many health experts indicate, however, that every one is different; thus, the number, severity and length of some of these symptoms can indicate that an individual is depressed.

TREATING DEPRESSION

Natural treatments of depression have recently received much attention (mainly to the emergence of St. John's wort), something that is very important because it gives depression sufferers one more tool with which to fight their condition. It is also important because diagnosed cases of depression are increasing in number each year. Accompanying the increase in depression cases and the emerging knowledge of its causes has been the rise of drug and other therapies in treating the disorder. This booklet will discuss the various treatments of depression in order to further teach the value of natural alternatives to treating the disorder.

STANDARD TREATMENTS FOR DEPRESSION

A wide variety of therapies have been employed to treat depression and other nervous disorders. When talking about standard treatments for depression, the two most important are psychotherapy and drug therapy. The following paragraphs address what these treatments entail.

Psychotherapy aims to resolve any underlying psychic conflicts that may be causing the depressed state, while giving emotional support to the patient. This usually involves seeing a psychiatrist and/or psychologist at regular intervals and may also include participation in support groups. Research does indicate that psychotherapy can be effective in aiding the sufferer to effectively deal with depression, but results are often sporadic and short lived.

Antidepressant drugs, on the other hand, directly affect the chemistry of the brain. For example, drugs affect neurochemicals such as monoamines, which are thought to have an important influence on depressed emotional states and moods. Other antidepressant drugs are thought to work by inhibiting the body's physiological inactivation of the monoamine transmitters. This results in the accumulation of these neurotransmitters in the brain and allows them to remain in contact with nerve cell receptors longer, thus aiding in elevating the mood of the patient. There are other drugs, called oxidase inhibitors, which interfere with the activity of monoamine oxidase, an enzyme known to be involved in the breakdown of two important brain chemicals, norepinephrine and serotonin.

While undergoing drug therapy is more favorable than continuing to suffer from depression, many individuals who take these medications experience very undesirable side effects. Uncomfortable physical side effects are among the biggest complaints about antidepressants. Many drug users suffer from sensations of nausea, bloating, indigestion, abdominal cramping and diarrhea, and other gastrointestinal discomforts. Dizziness is often a common complaint, as is dryness of the mouth, heart related problems, and many others. The following list gives a brief description of three of the most commonly prescribed antidepressant drugs.

STANDARD ANTIDEPRESSANT DRUGS

Prozac (Fluoxetine)

Prozac is a relatively new antidepressant that belongs to a drug class known as SSRIs, selective serotonin reuptake inhibitors. These increase the production of serotonin in the brain by inhibiting the serotonin reuptake process. Prozac was first introduced to the medical world in 1987 (other brand names of the drug have since appeared), and immediately took over the antidepressant market in this country. Sales have increased dramatically, topping the $1 billion mark last year. Its domination of the market is so widespread that the number of Prozac prescriptions is nearly twenty times that of all other standard antidepressants combined.

Though generally considered safe, Prozac has been linked to several undesired side effects—insomnia, anxiety, restlessness and others—indicating, in other words, that Prozac is too much of an "upper." Prozac has also been linked to different forms of destructive, if not bizarre, behavior. In fact, there are documented cases linking the drug to suicide. Other side effects of Prozac may include headaches, nausea, weight fluctuation, and dry mouth. In fact, one of Prozac's very attractive "attributes" is that of supposed weight loss (instead of the weight gain associated with other antidepressants). Research is showing, however, that despite initially losing weight after having started treatment, many of takers of Prozac eventually gain back what they weight lost and more if left on the drug long enough.

MAO Inhibitors

MAO (monoamine oxidase) inhibitors are the original antidepressant drugs, and help relieve depressive symptoms by inhibiting the enzyme monoamine oxidase, which is responsible for breaking down various chemical compounds in the brain, including serotonin. This lack of MAO allows for increased production of serotonin and norepinephrine, ultimately resulting in elevated mood levels. Because their primary effect is to stimulate rather than sedate, they can easily cause insomnia, the inability to focus, problems with coordination, as well as the typical side effects like dryness of mouth, gastrointestinal problems and dizziness. These side effects, however, are mild when compared to the possibility of severe reactions, possibly even death. Serious conditions, such as excessively high blood pressure and brain hemorrhage, can occur if the MAO inhibiting drug is taken with certain over-the-counter cold/cough remedies or certain foods, such as cheese, dried meats, wine and concentrated yeast products.

Tricyclic Antidepressants

Before the emergence of Prozac, tricyclic antidepressants were the most commonly prescribed for most cases of major depression and dysthemia. Their function is simply to encourage the activity of neurotransmitters in the brain and the nervous system and thereby decrease the occurrence of depressive symptoms. Despite being widely prescribed, these drugs too can cause a number of adverse side effects, including dryness of mouth, constipation and other gastrointestinal problems, dizziness, increased appetite (and weight gain), and blurred vision.

DEPRESSION—ALTERNATIVE TREATMENTS

Because depression often involves a complex mixture of severity, length, and mode of treatment, it is often a difficult decision for doctors and patients alike to decide how to treat the depression. Many practitioners and patients are reluctant to use antidepressant drugs because of associated side effects. It seems logical, then, that any additional forms of treatment with little risk, credible benefit, and moderate cost would be a useful addition to depression management.

Though the majority of depression sufferers employ antidepressant drugs to combat their condition, there are those who use more natural or "alternative" modes of treatment (though in this country their numbers are relatively few). The following descriptions examine the most common and effective supplements used in treating the various forms of depression.

St. John's Wort (Hypericum perforatum)

Of course, one of the most effective herbal remedies for depression is St. John's wort. Extracts of the herb have long been used in "folk" medicine for a range of symptoms and problems, including mood and depression disorders. Extracts of St. John's wort are licensed in Germany for the treatment of "anxiety and depressive and sleep disorders." In 1993, more than 2.7 million prescriptions of hypericum were given, making it one of the seven most popular prescriptions in Germany (Loese, et al 354). Other reports estimate hypericum prescriptions as constituting nearly half of the antidepressant market. In the past ten years, several randomized clinical trials have compared the effects of pharmaceutical preparations of hypericum with placebo and common antidepressants. Considering its apparent ability to relieve mild to moderate depression, and its extremely low rate of side effects, nearly all the studies favor the application of hypericum treatments for mild to moderate depression and other related disorders. These studies also show that the rates of occurrence of side effects are significantly lower than those of synthetic drugs, and at times, lower than those attributed to a placebo.

Is St. John's wort just a folk or alternative treatment for depression? While its popularity in this country is limited to the peripheral areas of health care, its use in Europe and other areas of the world would justify calling it mainstream.

St. John's wort, whose latin name is *Hypericum perforatum* (and to which we will also refer to as "hypericum") belongs to the family Hypericaceae, which consists of eight genuses and about 350 species. The herb has leaves that are whorled, gland-dotted, simple, and usually smooth-margined. Its flowers are five-petalled and yellow with many stamens, which are often united in bundles. It grows in many areas around the world, from Australia to Europe to the U.S. (it grows especially well in northern California and Oregon). Perhaps its somewhat peculiar name merits some explanation. The plant took on the name *St. John's wort* supposedly because it flowers around the time of St. John's Eve. The word *wort* comes from the Old English term *wyrt*, which means plant, herb or vegetable.

The first recorded use of St. John's wort occurred during the Crusades, mainly to treat battle wounds and enhance mental alertness. It was also used to treat the insane because of its effect on both the nervous system and brain. St. John's wort was even used to treat the supposed "possessions" and hallucinations of witches, as well as other forms of mental instability.

Contemporary research supports these uses, proving the herb's worth in aiding all types of topical wounds in their healing and recovery and in treating disorders of "mood and temperament." It is principally the latter—the treatment of depression ("mood and temperament")—that has prompted the writing of this booklet.

With the surfacing of several recent studies demonstrating St. John's wort's ability to treat depression while producing fewer side effects and having lower cost than standard antidepressant drugs, one may wonder why it is only now that Americans are being exposed to this medicinal plant. There are several probable reasons for this— our society's condescending attitude toward natural therapies, and the medical profession's unwillingness to trust the research indicating hypericum's ability to treat depression, are among them—though these are a topic for another book. The important thing to remember is that the research indicating hypericum's ability to treat depression is there (though there is still need for further investigation), and that consumers can turn to a mode of treatment that is as effective, costs less and produces fewer side effects than other synthetic antidepressant drugs.

How St. John's Wort Works

Though the research body concerning St. John's wort is increasing, there is still no conclusive data indicating exactly how the herb works. St. John's wort contains many chemical constituents, many of them recognized as possessing certain pharmacological properties. These chemical compounds include flavonols, flavanones, carotenoids, xanthones, phenolic carboxylic acids, sequiterpenes, monoterpenes and a number of dianthrones, among others.

One of the reasons St. John's wort is attracting so much interest is because of one of its compounds, hypericin. The journal *Photochemistry-Photobiology* recently published a review of hypericin and the structurally related hypocrellins, giving a favorable outline of the various recent breakthroughs in medicine using these two compounds. The review states:

> Hypocrellins and hypericins, structurally related plant pigments . . . are known photodynamic agents. This review summarizes certain significant advances in the photophysics, photochemistry and photobiology of these pigments in the last two years and discusses their prospects as novel therapeutic and diagnostic agents in the future . . . In particular, substantial progress has been made in both anticancer and antiviral applications (especially antihuman immunodeficiency virus) . . . The biomedical advances of hypocrellins and hypericins have been further promoted by significant progress in their chemical synthesis and the recent commercialization of hypericins. (Diwu, Z. 539)

Hypericin was isolated from St. John's wort in 1942 and has been thought of as the agent most responsible for giving St. John's wort its antidepressant capabilities. However, as previously mentioned, evidence for this remains inconclusive. But there are specific actions known to be demonstrated by hypericin. Among its many beneficial qualities is that of increasing blood flow to stressed tissue, thereby producing a tranquilizing effect. Hypericin also reduces the fragility of capillaries and enhances uterine muscle tone because of its ability to increase blood flow. Nearly all researchers are saying the same thing—that St. John's wort (and specifically hypericin) promises significant value to the medical world in overcoming depression and many other disorders.

RESEARCH CONCERNING ST. JOHN'S WORT AND DEPRESSION

In the last several years, there have been a number of studies comparing the effect of hypericum extract against placebo and standard antidepressants in regards to mild and moderate forms of major depression and their scope and severity of adverse side effects. One of the most recent studies exploring the effect of St. John's wort on depression, and which was instrumental in bringing the herb to the public's attention, revealed some fairly stunning results. *The British Medical Journal* (August 1996) published the results of the study, which consisted of twenty-three randomized trials, including a total of 1757 outpatients with mainly mild or moderately severe depressive disorders. Testing was conducted with 1) single preparations and combinations of extracts of the plant, 2) a placebo and 3) various standard drug treatments (imipramine, amitriptylin desipramin and others).

As just mentioned, the results were very promising. In all aspects of the study, hypericum extracts were shown to be "significantly superior" to placebo and similarly effective as standard antidepressants. The result worth noting is that there were more than twice the number, percentage-wise, of dropouts due to side effects from the standard drugs than those taking the hypericum extracts. Substantially more patients were taking hypericum extracts, and only fifty of them experienced side effects. Of the smaller group of patients using standard antidepressants, eighty-four experienced negative side effects. Dropout rates for the drugs were nearly double that of St. John's wort.

The scores on the Hamilton depression scale, which measures severity of one's depression, showed those taking hypericum treatments scored slightly higher than those taking the antidepressant and significantly higher than those taking the placebo (Linde, et al, 254). This study provides some firm ground for St. John's wort to stand on, both in sheer numbers and its quality of treatment.

Another contemporary study, carried out in 1995 by Witte, et. al, supports the findings of the Linde study. Carried out as a multicenter, placebo-controlled double-blind trial, this study used a hypericum preparation to treat ninety-seven outpatients. The course of the illness was assessed with the Hamilton Depression Scale, the vonZerssen Depressivity Scale and the Clinical Global Impression Scale. The authors of the study noted:

Treatment [with hypericum] resulted in an appreciable improvement in the symptoms of depression, and the seventy percent response rate (n=43) corresponded to that of chemical antidepressants. The preparation also showed an anxiolytic effect. The substance [hypericum] was extremely well tolerated, and no side effects were reported by any of the patients. (Witte, et al, 408-404)

Again, this study's findings correlate with those of the Linde and other studies in that treatment with hypericum is at least as effective as standard synthetic antidepressants and does not produce near the number of side effects.

The *Nursing Times* also reported on recent findings dealing with hypericum's effect on depression. Stating that psychiatric medications are notorious for their undesirable side effects and that the need for safer antidepressants is widely acknowledged, the magazine refers to a double-blind study done by G. Harrer and H. Sommer (published in *Phytomedicine*, 1994 (1): 3-8). The researchers used St. John's wort on 105 patients experiencing mild to moderate depression. These patients were aged twenty to sixty-four and had diagnoses of "neurotic depression or temporary depressive mood." Patients were divided into two groups and monitored over four weeks, with one group receiving 300 mg of hypericum extract three times daily and the other group receiving a placebo. All patients received psychiatric evaluations before the start of the study and after two and four weeks of treatment (Jackson, 49).

The results of the study support the findings of other recent studies dealing with hypericum and depression: 67 percent of the hypericum group responded positively to the treatment without any adverse side 'effects, whereas only 28 'percent of the placebo group displayed any improvement. Harrer and Sommer state that the patients treated were experiencing strictly mild forms of depression and, along with the results of other studies, suggest that hypericum treatment can be a very effective treatment for mild to moderate depression without severe side effects. The authors themselves even recommended that St. John's wort should be considered as a remedy of choice (Harrer, Sommer, 3-8).

These and other studies point to the strong possibility of using St. John's wort on a wide scale to treat various forms of depression. Many sufferers of depression are very concerned about side effects, but Linde's study suggests that St. John's wort's most valuable asset may be that it has few or no side effects. The authors do note, however, that more research is necessary, especially in determining the severity and nature of depression, length of treatment, treatment dosage, preparation of hypericum extracts, and occurrence of long-term side effects. Nevertheless, the results of this study and many others are extremely promising for the millions of those who suffer from various levels of major depression and dysthemia.

STUDIES OF ST. JOHN'S WORT'S EFFECTS ON DEPRESSION

Over the last twelve years or so, more than two dozen studies have been conducted comparing hypericum's effects on depression with that of placebos and other standard antidepressant drug therapies. When comparing these studies, several things stand out (many of these things have been discussed previously, but additional mention here emphasizes the broad scale and relative thoroughness of the studies). The following are some notes of interest.

- In several of the studies, the number of subjects who dropped out of the study nearly identical in the placebo group than in the group taking the hypericum extract (some were even higher). The number of dropouts from groups taking standard drug treatments in their respective studies was usually significantly higher than the hypericum groups. This is certainly a strong case for the argument that hypericum extracts cause few or no undesirable side effects, something that is of principal concern to most depression sufferers.
- Many of the studies note that the hypericum groups record much higher rates of patients who are "very much improved" and "no longer ill"; that is, they do not demonstrate sufficient symptomalogy under the various depression rating systems to qualify as depressed after they have been treated with hypericum. This indicates that hypericum's therapeutic activity is very potent—perhaps potent enough to completely relieve one of depression.
- Of particular interest are the results obtained from a study done by Vorbach, et al. Because most previous studies involving hypericum were carried out using subjects suffering only mild to moderate depression, the accepted use of hypericum for treating depression has been only for those in the mild to moderate range; it was not recommended for those suffering from severe major depression.

This study, however, showed hypericum outperforming imipramine (a standard antidepressant used for severe depression) when used on sufferers of severe depression. Of course, more studies should be done to corroborate these findings, but at the same time, given hypericum's very safe record and proven ability to fight moderate depression levels, it should not surprise us that it works for severe depression levels as well.

- Several studies show (as does commentary by the researchers) that hypericum seems to "build up" its effect, becoming more and more effective the longer it is used.
- All the researchers in these studies have recommended that hypericum be used as a viable option for treatment of mild to moderate depression because of its broad range of therapeutic activity, its relative lack of side effects and and excellent treatment record. (This is of special appeal to many because many of the researchers are trained health practitioners in standard medicine, not natural or herbal medicine, and thereby not necessarily "sympathetic" toward alternative health treatments).

OTHER NATURAL TREATMENTS FOR DEPRESSION

Besides St. John's wort, there are several other natural treatments for depression, including herbal and natural supplements, diet, exercise, and various others. If you are looking for treatment options other than the standard antidepressant drug, there are various types of health care professionals, including doctors of osteopathy, chiropractics, and naturopathy, that can recommend effective therapies employed to treat depression. Recently, St. John's wort and other herbal/nutritional supplements have entered the spotlight as the "hot" new treatments for depression and other related disorders. Some of these, including valerian, have been tested in several studies as a combination therapy with St. John's wort. Information on these complementary therapies follows.

Valerian Root (Valeriana officinalis)

Valerian has long been used to treat disorders of the nervous system, including depression, insomnia, and anxiety. Its sedative effects have been well documented. In fact, it was listed in this country's two major medicinal registers, the *U.S. Pharmacopeia* and the *U.S. Formulary* as a tranquilizing agent. In addition, it has been shown to combat hormonal instabilities like those common in premenstrual syndrome and postmenopausal stages. These hormonal instabilities can have an intense effect on the brain and nervous system.

As mentioned previously, valerian has the ability to reduce insomnia and promote high-quality sleep. It has a relaxing effect on smooth muscle, and inhibits the processes of the nervous system, thereby promoting a calm feeling and eventually a deeper, more restful sleep. Recent research indicates that besides being very helpful in improving sleep quality, valerian does not produce the side effects of sluggishness or grogginess common to the tranquilizer-like drugs used to promote sleep.

5-HTP (5-Hydroxytryptophan)

5-HTP, an emerging treatment for depression and related conditions, is the raw material by which the body makes serotonin, one of the key substances that maintains mood levels in the brain. 5-HTP can be formed by the body from tryptophan, a naturally occurring amino acid. Though known for years as a player in serotonin production, it is only recently that American doctors and consumers are focusing on 5-HTP as a treatment for depression and other mood disorders. Its antidepressant properties, however, are fast being recognized as one of the most powerful and safe methods to fighting depression

Researchers began investigating 5-HTP and its possible therapeutic capabilities in the 1960s. Early on in these studies, it was discovered that 5-HTP was quickly converted into serotonin. But the lack of research only led these researchers to wonder about the safety of 5-HTP, its application for humans, and what possible side effects its use could produce.

Consequently, studies were initiated to investigate how 5-HTP worked, and whether or not it was safe to use. Some of the first were conducted in Japan. One of these, conducted in 1970, involved patients suffering from either unipolar or bipolar (the most severe form of depression) depression. Within approximately two weeks, more than 50 percent of the patients experienced some sort of improvement in their symptoms; when the four-week trial was concluded, almost three-fourths of the patients indicated they had experienced either complete relief of symptoms or at least significant improvement (Sano, 1424).

Another study, one of the most thorough and impressive of the Japanese studies, involved both male and female patients whose depression levels were determined to be moderate to severe. The patients were given multiple daily doses for approximately three weeks; the majority of the subjects experienced improvement in their symptoms and reported only minimal side effects (Nakajima, et al., 223-30).

There have been numerous studies since the pioneer studies carried out by the Japanese. One of the most controlled and convincing, conducted in 1991, was conducted by Swiss researchers who compared 5-hydroxytryptophan to a popular SSRI antidepressant, Luvox. Results were taken at the two-, four-, and six-week marks. Overall, the results favored 5-hydroxytryptophan. Its overall degree of improvements was better than that of Luvox (61 percent to 56 percent), 5-HTP worked faster than Luvox, and a lower side effect rate was reported among 5-HTP users than with Luvox (Poldinger, et al., 53-81).

There are numerous studies examining 5-HTP's abilities to not only fight depression, but also combat disorders that often accompany (or are a result of) depression. These include eating disorders, obesity, sleep disorders, migraines, chronic fatigue, autoimmune diseases, and others. For more information on these and a more complete discussion on depression and the seemingly amazing therapeutic properties of 5-HTP, read Michael Murray's book, *5-HTP: The Natural Way to Overcome Depression, Obesity, and Insomnia,* published by Bantam Books.

Kava (Piper methysticum)

This plant, whose common name comes from various South Pacific island cultures, was often used by these same cultures for promoting sleep and as a relaxant. Kava is also noted for its muscle relaxing abilities, a trait valuable in relieving anxiety and agitation and promoting deeper sleep. Like valerian, kava is effective as a tranquilizer in promoting sleep, and does so without the "hangover" symptoms common to other standard sleeping drugs. Kava is also used for other conditions of the nervous system, including anxiety and mild forms of depression.

Hops

Hops has long been used as a mood stabilizer and natural sedative. In 18th-century Europe, field workers involved in harvesting hops could rarely work a full day because they became so fatigued from working with the plant. Like other nervine herbs, hops has long been recognized as being effective in promoting muscle relaxation and more restful sleep, relieving other symptoms of insomnia and stabilizing moods. One reason for these nervine properties may be the plant's high B-vitamin content. The various B vitamins play a crucial role in maintaining various body systems; a deficiency in one or more of these vitamins can cause a plethora of ailments directly related to the nervous system, including sleep disorders, depression, and anxiety (see section in this chapter on vitamin/mineral link to improving depression).

Amino Acids

Amino acids are now recognized as essential to overall health. Their role in treating mood disorders is also becoming more well known. Certain amino acids, including L-tryptophan (see discussion on 5-HTP), L-tyrosine and L-phenylalanine, aid the body in producing amines, neurotransmitters that serve the brain and nervous system. If the body is deficient in these amino acids, then the obvious consequence is a drop in neurotransmitter function and ultimately a "drop" in mood. These amino acids are useful in treating the carbohydrate craving of SAD sufferers (discussed in the SAD section of this chapter), and in raising the levels of serotonin, dopamine and norepinephrine, probably the three most crucial compounds involved in controlling mood levels.

Vitamin/Mineral Therapy

More and more research is indicting certain vitamin and mineral deficiencies as a principal cause of depression and other nervous disorders. Of particular concern are the B vitamins. Deficiencies of vitamin B6 has been linked to depression sufferers, including new mothers whose B6 levels are abnormally low. Exactly why a B6 deficiency causes or exaggerates a depression episode is not exactly known. But the numbers point to its being a factor: nearly 20 percent of all depression sufferers are also suffering from a B6 deficiency. Those taking oral contraceptives, other synthetic drugs, or even ingesting high levels of caffeine, are also known to have depleted B6 levels. Other B vitamins like B3, B12 and B1 are necessary for other physiological processes, including the production of essential amino acids, a central factor in controlling one's psychiatric state.

In considering vitamin deficiencies, it is readily apparent that vitamin C plays a principal role in mood and nervous system management. Taking vitamin C with bioflavonoids has been shown to considerably aid in the synthesizing of norepinephrine and serotonin, two of the brain's major neurotransmitters. Flavonoids, which are nutrients not produced by the body, are found naturally in the rinds of citrus fruits, green peppers, tomatoes, broccoli, cherries and other commonly eaten foods. Bioflavonoids help vitamin C be assimilated more easily, thereby enhancing the vitamin's mood elevating capabilities.

Ginkgo biloba

Ginkgo biloba is a popular herb used to enhance mental clarity and circulation in the brain and extremities. Traditionally, ginkgo has been used in China and surrounding areas for various purposes for literally thousands of years; its main purposes in the Chinese medical repertoire was for enhancing brain function and improving respiratory health.

Currently, there is a large body of legitimate scientific research indicating that ginkgo does indeed improve circulation to the brain (and peripheral areas of the body), thereby enhancing mental alertness and mood and giving a sense of more energy. Thus, ginkgo is widely used in Europe and other countries (and is becoming increasingly popular in the U.S.) for treating mild to moderate depression.

Who does ginkgo most help? Well, the answer to this question isn't exactly clear, but research does give us some indication that it may inhibit the age-related loss of serotonin receptors; in other words, older persons suffering from depression (which may be caused by the "natural" loss of serotonin receptors in the brain) may especially benefit from taking ginkgo. Another study focusing on patients who had tried therapy with synthetic drugs but had not experienced any relief showed impressive results. Fifty percent of those patients given ginkgo experienced successful results while only ten percent of the placebo group showed improvement. This study is significant for two reasons: first, ginkgo was able to benefit persons who had already tried standard antidepressant drugs but experienced no relief; second, the success rate of the ginkgo therapy was clearly superior to that of the placebo success rate.

What about side effects of ginkgo therapy? Considering all of the research, side effects associated with taking ginkgo are essentially nonexistent. Though ginkgo may not help everyone who suffers from depression (as is the case with any therapy), it is generally accepted by most health experts that ginkgo can provide a natural and safe alternative to standard antidepressant drugs.

Light Therapy and SAD

In treating SAD, the knowledge that lack of light causes or at least contributes the disorder has made phototherapy, or light therapy, a natural choice of remedy. Studies done on light therapy shows that it is usually effective in relieving most of the symptoms of depression. It seems to do this by encouraging the production of serotonin in the brain, one of the principal agents involved in determining the state of one's mood. Sunlight also provides the body with vitamin D, needed by the body for proper assimilation of calcium. Studies suggest that problems with the absorption of vitamin D and calcium correlate with the onset of depression, most notably in the form of SAD.

Phototherapy has been used on people who work graveyard shifts or shifts that go partially through the night. It has also been used to treat travelers, most of whom suffer from jet lag. Researchers have shown that phototherapy is effective when combined with hypericum therapy. The study shows that the hypericum extract used on SAD sufferers was very effective in helping the SAD patients overcome a majority of the depression symptoms (as effective as treating major depression shown in other studies). Results from this study also showed hypericum to be as effective, if not more so, than phototherapy, the popular choice for most mental health care practitioners. The researchers also note that hypericum therapy might well become the most popular mode of treatment because many patients regard phototherapy as too time consuming.

Exercise

Exercise can prove extremely valuable in overcoming depression. Several studies indicate that exercise alone can dramatically improve one's mood levels and their ability to handle internal and external stress. Needless to say, the general health benefits of exercise do not need to be emphasized. One recent study found that depressed subjects who increased their participation in physical activities (sports, exercise activities, etc.) experienced a significant decrease in feelings of depression, malaise, and related ailments like insomnia.

THE MISDIAGNOSIS OF DEPRESSION

One relatively new and disturbing trend in the study of depression is that too often a person showing depression-like symptoms is automatically diagnosed as having depression, when in fact it is a reversible physical disorder that is "causing" or encouraging the onset of the depression. This, of course, raises several disturbing questions, among them "Why are people being misdiagnosed?" and "What about the undiscovered physical condition?" We can preface the answer to each question by noting that recent studies have shown that initial treatments for various forms of depression and mood disorders (both prescription drug therapy and psychotherapy) are increasingly showing lower and lower success rates. Why is this important? If we accept the idea that the depression can be a symptom of another physical ailment, then treating the underlying physical disorder, not prescribing antidepressants, is the ideal way of relieving depressive symptoms.

In response to the first inquiry about why people are being misdiagnosed, we must first determine if misdiagnosis really is a problem in the treatment of depression. There are a number of studies that strongly suggest that physical disorders play an important role in the development of and/or mimicking of a psychiatric disorder. A 1979 study of 2090 depressed subjects showed that 43 percent of these were suffering from one or more physical illnesses, 46 percent of which were not diagnosed at the time of the original diagnosis of depression. A significant number of these patients were suffering from a major physical disorder that was directly causing their symptoms of depression (Koranyi, 1979). A 1982 study provided strikingly similar results. The study consisted of 215 patients who were sent to a psychiatry specialist for additional evaluation of the initial diagnosis of depression. The study's numbers are disconcerting; 41 percent of the patients were inaccurately diagnosed and 24 percent of the original diagnoses were changed, either from physical to psychiatric disorders or vice versa.

So, is misdiagnosis a major problem? Studies indicate a definite "yes." The previously discussed studies and others suggest that a principal cause of improper diagnosis is that of a physical ailment presenting itself with symptoms akin to depression and mood disorders. In fact, Gold points out that medical professionals, both mental and medical, perform relatively poorly in diagnosing a physical ailment if the ailment is accompanied by psychiatric symptoms (Gold 96).

The Relationship of Depression and Physical Disorders

In response to questions concerning the undiscovered physical condition, it is becoming more and more apparent that there are a number of other conditions—including physical disorders, medications and drug/alcohol use—that produce symptoms similar or equal to those of the various forms of depression. In fact, psychiatric symptoms are commonly the first showing of some reversible illness of a physical, not psychological or emotional, nature.

The presence of psychiatric symptoms that suggest a state of depression or mood disorder, coupled with the the way a health practitioner approaches the diagnosis, may be the primary causes of misdiagnosis. A doctor (be it a general practitioner, specialist, psychiatrist or other) may exhibit a simple lack of knowledge, the inability to deal with physical illness, a lag in training programs, a lack of continuing education, or an unwillingness to incorporate new information into the treatment regimens. We should not hasten to malign physicians, however. A 1980 study by Klein and associates suggests that although there certainly are errors in diagnosis, there are multiple reasons, most not fault of the practitioner, that lead to misdiagnosis (Gold, 96).

At least two studies shed light on reasons for misdiagnosis. Researchers McIntyre and Romano found that less than 35 percent of the polled psychiatrists give their subjects any sort of physical exam (which could include simple questions as to other symptoms not related to depression, and/or use of other medications, alcohol or drugs). Their study shows that even less of these doctors felt somewhat unable to perform a thorough physical. And these numbers may be even greater. Gold states that most mental health practitioners consult with the subject's general practitioner, specialist, gynecologist, etc. in place of performing the physical themselves—though this is, admittedly, better than nothing (Gold, 97). As stated before, both medical and psychiatric professionals show overall poor numbers in correctly diagnosing a physical ailment when it is accompanied by symptoms of depression and other psychiatric disturbances.

What all this essentially means is that, for one reason or another, there is certain information that the health care practitioner either is not privy to or lax in obtaining, and therefore, unable to use in successfully determining the cause of the patient's symptoms. And this leads to the practitioner more easily "placing" the patient into an area of his of her specialty or orientation, which finally leads to "a distortion and misperception of the client and his or her sometimes obvious physical illness" (Gold, 97).

The Common Culprits

While there are many disorders that border on the fine line between physical and mental health (thus making a correct diagnosis difficult), there also are several others that truly present themselves solely as psychiatric in nature. Upon correct identification and treatment of the physical disorder, the symptoms of depression/mood disturbances usually clear up without any treatment for the depression. There are other physical disorders, such as diabetes and others listed below, that present themselves at least partially with symptoms of a psychiatric nature, and when successfully treated, end in a partial clearing of the psychiatric symptomatology (Gold 97-98). The following are several of the most common physical ailments that present themselves as being either completely or partially psychiatric in nature, and whose presence either accentuates the depressive state or is the sole cause.

DIABETES (Diabetes Mellitus)

Studies have shown that diabetes can manifest itself as major depression—its symptoms meet the diagnostic criteria for such (Hall, 1981). Just the stress it puts on the body because of fluctuating blood sugar levels can essentially wreak havoc on the liver, kidneys and endocrine system.

HYPERTHYROIDISM/HYPOTHYROIDISM

Hyperthyroidism can mimic the symptoms of several mental disorders, including panic disorder, mania, neurosis and depression.

Hypothyroidism can also resemble psychiatric disturbances—in fact a form of hypothyroidism can often show symptoms that concur with the DSM-IV criteria for major depression (Gold, 104).

VITAMIN DEFICIENCIES

There are numerous studies that indict vitamin (and mineral) deficiencies as principal culprits in the mimicking of depression. These deficiencies are especially common to the B vitamins, and include vitamin B12, niacin, folic acid, folate, and zinc. The symptoms of these deficiencies are varied; they include paranoia, irritability, apathy, schizophrenia, fatigue, depression, weight loss and appetite loss, among others.

HEAVY METAL POISONING

The number of heavy metal poisonings has risen in recent years. The overconsumption of these metals occurs chiefly from high levels of exposure or, more simply, ingesting. The most common metals involved in poisonings are lead, mercury, manganese, zinc, magnesium, copper, arsenic and aluminum. Elevated levels of any of these in the body can cause a form of "brain allergy," thereby producing symptoms similar to those of psychiatric and mental illness, namely major depression.

HYPOGLYCEMIA

Many people suffer from a hypoglycemic condition that produces symptoms nearly identical to those of various mental disorders such as depression. The symptoms are usually exaggerated by the inconsistencies in the body's blood-sugar levels and overall difficulty in proper glucose assimilation. Such a condition causes a definite "low" in physical energy levels and ultimately a "low" in mental and emotional levels as well.

DRUG/ALCOHOL USE

The very nature of illicit drugs and alcohol should suggest that their use (and abuse) could easily result in symptoms of mental disorders. What is of interest is that many studies have repeatedly shown that prescription drugs are a principal cause of depression-like symptoms. *Prevention's New Encyclopedia of Common Diseases* quotes the *Journal of the American Geriatric Society*, stating, "Drugs, either prescribed by a physician or taken independently, are often responsible for the development of depression, the aggravation of a preexisting depression, or the production of depression-like symptoms . . ." (233).

Gold points out that it is very easy for symptoms of drug users to mimic a wide array of psychiatric disorders, including major depression. He also notes that it is essential for the health care provider to follow strict and proper testing for determining the extent of drug use, intoxication and withdrawal to conclusively rule out or consider psychiatric disorders as the cause of the symptomalogy (Gold, 101).

Drug use and depression is also a topic among the elderly. A large majority of elderly people in our country take multiple prescription drugs for a variety of ailments, and most of these medications cause one or more adverse side effects. Combining medications can be detrimental for the person, both in efficacy of the medications and in the possible creation of additional side effects.

Also of interest here is the topic of alcohol abusers and the use of St. John's wort. As discussed later, there is certainly a strong link between alcohol abuse and the occurrence of depression. While studies suggest that hypericum is effective in treating alcohol-induced depression, what needs to be realized is that the eradication of the substance abuse (either alcohol, illicit drug or prescription drug) will at least partially, and possibly completely, the symptoms of depression and other mood regularities.

The following are several, but certainly not all, types of prescription drugs that can mimic symptoms of major depression.

- anti-inflammatories (Naprosyn)
- birth control pills (and other hormonal medicines)
- hypertension medications (Apresoline)
- heart medications
- sleeping medications (Valium)

TUMORS (CANCER)

Various forms of malignant tumors have been known to create depressive symptoms, even before physical signs of the tumor appear. Carcinoid tumors often secrete dopamine, histamine, corticotropin, and serotonin, all substances that can have a profound effect on the brain and other systems of the body (Gold, 99).

NUTRITIONAL HABITS

Recently the idea that what we eat can have a profound effect on our brain chemistry and other seemingly non-related body systems has gained more widespread acceptance in the medical community. The connection between nutritional deficiencies, food sensitivities and allergies, and overall poor dietary habits is demanding more investigation in its role in promoting and/or encouraging depression and other related nervous disorders. In fact, research indicates that the most common symptoms, or side effects, of food allergies are headaches, fatigue and depression. Digestion of offending substances causes the body to react as if being "invaded" by foreign allergens, in turn causing other body systems to react. Brain chemistry is inevitably affected, many times displaying its effects in an episode of mood or nervous disorders.

OTHER DISORDERS MANIFESTING DEPRESSIVE SYMPTOMS
• hyperadrenalism/hypoadrenalism
• cancer
• mononucleosis
• hepatitis (all forms)
• multiple sclerosis

What to Do?

The idea that disorders and conditions separate from depression, namely physical in nature, can completely or partially "cause" depression should ring true to any sensible person. In the introduction to a compilation of articles on depression, Dr. Frederic Flach stresses the idea that depression is not necessarily its own illness; rather, it is a symptom (or group of symptoms) that the body enacts when dealing with other stresses and disturbances. He states:

> Early on [in his career], I could appreciate the complexity of depression, in which psychological, environmental, and biologic factors all played significant etiological roles. . . . In this context, I reformulated my own concept of what depression is—and what it is not. Being depressed, per se, is neither a weakness nor an illness. Rather, depression is the way healthy human beings respond to certain stresses . . . Depression can be viewed as an illness when it is not recognized and acknowledged, when it gets out of hand and overwhelms a client, when it persists, and—most important—when the individual cannot recover from an episode on his or her own. (Flach xiii-xiv)

Naturopathic and holistic-minded physicians have always stressed the notion that many of today's diseases are not technically diseases—they are often the symptoms the body produces in response to some other deeper, underlying disorder. Symptoms disappear when the underlying cause is taken care of.

How, then, does one go about identifying the possible physical disorders affecting his or her depression? Dr. Gold recommends that a person undergo a complete physical, neurological and endocrinological examination by a professional trained in both psychiatry and internal medicine. Hopefully, these examinations will reveal other conditions that could be the origin of the depressive state (Gold, 108). From there, a complete regimen involving physical, emotional and psychiatric aid can be implemented. Simple lifestyle changes, such as diet alterations and increased physical activity, can have profound changes on the severity, length and frequency of depression episodes. And using natural supplements such as hypericum extract instead of a more harsh synthetic antidepressant can aid in the eventual recovery of depression.

(NOTE: Mark Gold, M.D., provides an excellent source for more complete information on underlying causes of and misdiagnosis of depression in his article "The Risk of Misdiagnosing Physical Illness as Depression," found in *Managing Depression*, published by Hatherleigh Press.)

CONCLUSION

Depression can be a devastating disorder; however, it can be successfully overcome through natural and lifestyle changes, allowing for a normal and productive life. Research abounds indicating that depression is a largely misdiagnosed and mistreated disorder, and that there are a number of "alternative" therapies—including St. John's wort, valerian, 5-HTP, and light therapy—that can successfully and safely overcome depression. If one is looking for alternatives to standard drug treatments, and is willing to make basic lifestyle changes, the result can be a happy, normal life void of the shadow of depression.

Bibliography

Acosta, E.P., Fletcher, C.V. "Agents for Treating Human Immunodeficiency Virus Infection." *American Journal of Hospital Pharmacy* 51 (1994): 2251-67.

Andreoni, A., et al. "Laser Photosensitization of Cells by Hypericin." *Photochemistry-Photobiology* 59(5) (1996): 529-33.

Diwu, Z. "Novel Therapeutic and Diagnostic Applications of Hypocrellins and Hypericins." *Photochemistry-Photobiology* 61(6) (1989): 529-39.

Encyclopedia Britannica, (8) 1993: 21.

Flach, Frederic. "Introduction." In *The Hatherleigh Guide to Managing Depression.* New York: Hatherleigh Press, 1996.

Flynn, Rebecca, M.S. and Roest, Mark. *Your Guide to Standardized Herbal Products.* Prescott, Az.: One World Press, 1995.

Gold, Mark S., M.D. "The Risk of Misdiagnosing Physical Illness as Depression." In *The Hatherleigh Guide to Managing Depression.* New York: Hatherleigh Press, 1996.

Hall, R. C. W., et al. "Unrecognized Physical Illness Prompting Psychiatric Admission: A Prospective Study." *American Journal of Psychiatry* 138 (1981): 629-635.

Hänsgen, K. D., Vesper, J., Ploch, M. "Multicenter Double-Blind Study Examining the Antidepressant Effectiveness of the Hypericum Extract LI 160." *Journal of Geriatric Psychiatry and Neurology* 7 (1994): S15-S18.

Harrer, G., Hübner, W.D., Podzuweit, H. "Effectiveness and Tolerance of the Hypericum Extract LI 160 Compared to Maprotiline: A Multicenter Double-Blind Study." *Journal of Geriatric Psychiatry and Neurology* 7 (1994): S24-S28.

Harrer, G., H. Sommer. "Treatment of Mild/Moderate Depression with Hypericum." *Phytomedicine* 1 (1994): 3-8.

Hudson, J.B., Lopez-Bazzocchi, I., Towers, G.H. "Antiviral Activities of Hypericin." *Antiviral—Res.* 15 (1992): 101-12.

Jackson, Adam. "Herbal Help for Depression." *Nursing Times* 9 (1995): 49.

Johnson, D., et al. "Effects of Hypericum Extract LI 160 Compared with Maprotiline on Resting EEG and Evoked Potentials in 24 Volunteers." *Journal of Geriatric Psychiatry and Neurology* 7 (1994): S44-S46.

Journal of Association of Nurses Aids Care. Jan-Feb. (1995): 225.

Koranyi, E.K. "Morbidity and Rate of Undiagnosed Physical Illness in a Psychiatric Clinic Population." *Archives of General Psychiatry* 36 (1979): 414-449.

Krylov, A., Ibatov A. "The Use of an Infusion of St. John's Wort in the Combined Treatment of Alcoholics with Peptic Ulcer and Chronic Gastritis." *Vrach.-Delo.* Feb.-Mar. (1993): 146-8.

Lavie, G. et al. "Hypericin as an Inactivator of Infectious Viruses in Blood Components." *Transfusion* 35 (1995): 392-400.

Linde, et al. "St. John's Wort for Depression—An Overview and Meta-Analysis of Randomised Clinical Trials." *The British Medical Journal* 313 (1996): 253.

Lohse, et al. *Arzneiverordnungreport* 1994: 354.

Martinez, B., et al. "Hypericum in the Treatment of Seasonal Affective Disorders." *Journal of Geriatric Psychiatry and Neurology* 7 (1994): S29-33

Miskovsky, P., et al. "Subcellular Distribution of Hypericin in Human Cancer

Cells." *Photochem-Photobiol* 62 (1995): 546-9.

Nakajima,T., Y. Kudo, and Z. Kaneko, "Clinical evaluation of 5-hydroxytryptophan as an antidepressant drug," *Folia Psychiatrica et Neurologica Japonica* 32 (1978): 223-30.

Poldinger, W., B. Calanchini,and W. Schwartz, " A functional-dimensional approach to depression: Serotonin deficiency as a target syndrome in a comparison of 5-HTP and fluvoxamine," *Psychopathology* 24(1991): 53-81.

Ritchason, Jack. *The Little Herb Encyclopedia.* Pleasant Grove, UT: Woodland Publishing, 1994.

Ross, C.E. and Hayes, D. "Exercise and psychological well-being in the community," American Journal of Epidemiology, 127 (1988): 762-71.

Sano, I. "L-5-hydroxytryptophan therapy," *Folia Psychiatrica et Neurologica Japonica* 26(1972): 1424.

Schulz, H., Jobert, M. "Effects of hypericum extract on the sleep EEG in older volunteers." *The Journal of Geriatric Psychiatry and Neurology* 7 (1994): S39-43.

Science. 254 (1991): 522.

VanderWerf, Q.M., et al. "Hypericin: a new laser phototargeting agent for human cancer cells." *Lanryngyscope* 106 (1996): 479-83.

Vorbach, E., Hübner, W., Arnoldt, K. "Effectiveness and Tolerance of the Hypericum Extract LI 160 in Comparison with Imipramine: Randomized Double-Blind Study with 135 Outpatients." *Journal of Geriatric Psychiatry and Neurology* 7 (1994): S19-23.

Wagner, H. and S. Bladt. "Pharmaceutical Quality of Hypericum Extracts." *Journal of Geriatric Psychiatry and Neurology* 7 (1994): S65-68.

Witte, B., et al. "Treatment of Depressive Symptoms with a High Concentration of Hypericum Preparation." *Fortschr. Med.* 113 (1995): 404-8.

Woelk, H., Burkard, G., Grünwald, J. "Benefits and Risks of the Hypericum Extract LI 160: Drug Monitoring Study with 3250 Patients." *Journal of Geriatric Psychiatry and Neurology* 7 (1994): S34-38.